CW01472065

Intermittent Fasting

for women

Sophia Omad Brown

Legal & Disclaimer

Upon using the contents and information contained in this book, you agree that the author is not in any way responsible for damages, costs, and expenses, including any legal fees potentially resulting from the application of any of the information provided by this book.

This disclaimer applies to any loss, damages or injury caused by the use and application, whether directly or indirectly, of any advice or information presented, whether for breach of contract, tort, negligence, personal injury, criminal intent, or under any other cause of action.

You agree to accept all risks of using the information presented inside this book.

You agree that during the course of reading this book, where appropriate and/or necessary, you shall consult a professional (including but not limited to your doctor, attorney, or financial advisor or such other advisor as needed) before using any of the suggested remedies, techniques, or information in this book.

All you need to know

about Intermittent Fasting.

The secrets and the powers.

Contents

Introduction

The urgent calls to shed off body fat has led dieticians and physicians to yet approve another strategy called Intermittent Fasting.

What did we use to have?

Much before this method, all we had was packs of hard calisthenics that end up making you feel like somebody battered your body and soul with hammers. You feel so tired sometimes that going to work that day is a mission-impossible. that's still simple.

It may get so worse that you can't walk, talk or even eat, all you can do is breathe and watch. Of course, you may feel excited since you'll feel the effect if done consistently, but there's no two-way to say it tires you, it really tires.

The next and probably easier method we have witnessed is to be on medication. It's true that you can shed off a good deal of fats by taking certain drugs. Many people do it and it worked for them.

But that's where the problem begins; it doesn't work for everyone.

Due to our different body systems, we have different allergies. That's why your doctor would keep asking you when considering drug recommendation, 'are you allergic to septrin?' 'are you allergic to this and to that?'.

All because what works for your husband or your twin sister may not work perfectly for you. Your system is exclusively for you.

Unfortunately, most of these drugs are not recommended by experts, so nobody can even help you see what's best and what is next for you, you get to do it yourself.

Since we are not experts, what do you expect? We end up exposing ourselves to dangers and drug abuse. In fact, you may be saying 'hi' to cancer that way.

Even at those times your drugs are recommended by experts, you still stand a danger of something, side effects. Drugs like this usually have a negative effect that can be, you know, disastrous.

You use them and you just realize some cells are dead, you lose taste and interest in meals, including your favorite. Some got lean than they ever hoped and many don't feel as excited as you used to be again.

That's just some out of the hundreds of possible complications. So get in a ward and chat a doctor, every single one of them tells you drug isn't your first option.

The near alternative to these ones is the diet ration method. Actually, doctors name this a lot and it seems to work wonders. All you need do is feed on a particular ration of food daily.

Usually, that's smaller than what you used to, and also awkward. You don't choose what you eat anymore, your dish timetable must be approved by your doctors first.

They tell you what you should eat and what you shouldn't, they tell you when to eat, what proportion and what not to ever. Maybe that's not very bad, but to me, I call it horrible.

Just how would I live only by what someone tells me? Why do I have to see some dietician every single second I feel like adding something to my own dietary table?

They measure the size of salt, rice, milk and …oh is this really sane? You know how it feels to see someone eating what you love and all you can do is watch because your doctor says no. It hurts really. As it happens most times, why do I have to leave what I love eating all because I want to lose some pounds, don't I really have a better option?

I must confess to you; I am not the only with those crazy questions.

While I was in the waiting hall the first time at the dieticians to lament that I hate living on no eggs, I got into talk with many of those waiting too, and guess what, we all came to protest our diets!

Didn't you ask these questions? Did it really work for you? Perhaps it works for some people, but I feel the percentage of protestants has risen so high that our physicians were left with no choice but to suggest and approve a newer, easier and much more comfortable method for us.

We call it INTERMITTENT FASTING.

Intermittent fasting is one of the biggest cures you can ever find yourself without spending a penny today.

Ever since I began to try it, I can tell you boldly that I have lost more pounds than other methods. I have gained muscles too. and the most amazing of all, I control my body weight with ease.

Without stressing my life out, risking drug abuse or cutting my delicacies (I am an awesome cook); I stopped being the woman that presses the car down with her weight every time she enters.

Now, I know when I am getting out of shape and I can, without spending my life as the dietician pleases get back into shape!

Intermittent Fasting is the Revised Standard Version of Fasting. I so much love this method that I am conducting researches, giving talks, starting a health spa and writing books on it.

Why do you need to lose some pounds?

Before I fully discuss details of how you can use intermittent fasting to lose some pounds, let's talk about why you need to lose those pounds.

You know, many of us look pretty cool in a medium shape, not-fat, not-thin stature. Actually, that's the smart stature. But it is too hard to maintain that kind of shape.

Eat a bit too much or take some reckless meals and you'll find yourself fatter than anyone in the banking hall. Break the food cycle too and you will suspect the person in the mirror of AIDS if you are not cautious. That's how difficult it is to maintain a stable body shape.

For some people, it goes far beyond maintaining body shape. They have grown excessively fat sometimes due to some genetic traits and sometimes how they live and what they eat. Either ways, they grew fat and they grew problems.

Excess Fats is poison to you. Today, many people can no longer breathe properly, some can't stride up or down a staircase, while some are simply too big enter vehicles.

Well, no matter how big you are, something can always be done, trust me, at 300 pounds, I was getting bigger than a vehicle!

For some people, they don't have health complications yet, but yes, they really do feel out of place. Some researchers recently discovered an amusing fact. They said the number of people becoming unhappy keeps rising on a daily basis. Many people feel very happy and confident when they are in their rooms.

You feel absolutely fine when preparing to hit the street and get some money, or probably catch up your friends en route party. But wait till these people meet their colleagues or probably friends who have something they don't, something simply goes missing inside their heart.

They would laugh about how slim and sexy they looked in her new dress and they would all boast about their curvy shape, right in front of you who look round like a full sack of black beans.

You sure weren't there target, but, you'd feel a ting of jealously or desire and you'll find yourself moody. It's worse when you're their target.

Heaven knows who on mother earth inspired men to start this wild hunt for slim girls with curvy waists too. But the girls aren't making a thing easier, they all want heavily fit men who seem to have all of the strength.

The quest for a gracefully slender body shape and an awesome fitness is now the biggest thorn in the heart of every one. So, both genders find themselves in a frenzied race for a smarter look.

Much beyond the immediate admiration, I bet you want everyone who meet you at 50 to tell you 'you look 27', not '77'.

That's one other magic losing some pounds and keeping yourself in shape can help you perform.

So, congratulations for laying your hands on the perfect guide to the simplest, easiest and most practicable method of keeping yourself in shape.

Why should you choose INTERMITTENT FASTING and why should you take me serious?

a. Well, Intermittent Fasting is still the easiest way to lose pounds, I say you confirm that at your Physician's.

b. You are not clamped to dietary constrictions, meal timetable and zany rations.

c. You don't lose your favorite meal just to lose pounds.

d. You don't get to see anyone just because you are adding something to your own food.

e. Other methods may not work for everyone, not this!

f. It is much easier and comfortable to control your own weight yourself.

g. And finally, I was getting bigger than a vehicle and at 26, now at 27 I looked like 19, does that say something?

Get yourself your favorite drink. Don't spill it on this book or on your phone out of over-excitement, or I am going to be very very mad at you. You did that? Let me see you laugh, great. I think you are laughing out your overweight already. Let's go!

Intermittent Fasting for Women

Chapter 1: Benefits of Intermittent Fasting

So, we'd better begin with the benefits. Let's tell our ears and eyes and body some of the amazing benefits in stock for them if they accept intermittent fasting. After all, we fast, they fast too, and they deserve to know why.

First thing you need to write in your mind before you even begin is that 'this isn't going to be easy but yes, we need this'. If you can make your brain and body understand that you all need it together, It'll be real fun to play with food.

You may spend the whole day with a vacant stomach and you won't even hear any organ scream because your everybody inside you is really ready for it.

Let me make a prediction. Sometimes, you are going to feel tired and weak, and bored and upset and you just want to break the rules. I know already alright? So relax, you can always return to this book and listen to me again.

Remember I was getting bigger 310 but today I am a very smart lady. Let me hear you yell to your body to 'let's do this again!' Yo, repeat that!

Warn your body that it'd better adjust too, or you might have to sit in an open truck driving round the city since no car survives your size.

Now seriously, you should train your body so much that if you find yourself among those glutton friends in a food competition and it's your fasting day, all your part in the game is just the referee and an excited audience, laughing at them and chanting scores.

If I were you, I probably would be asking myself something now first; if my body is ready to fight this long food battle, then my body is sure it's getting something at the end.

What's my body getting? Just losing fats? Well, you will be surprised to learn that that's a sip of the benefit ocean.

I have been at the health spa with women as plump as elephant or around that size and you know, the main reason most of them, including me wanted Intermittent fasting was to shed off these surplus meats. But thanks to our sessions with those awesome doctors, you will soon find out we're all in for more.

Apart from the benefits the doctors mentioned, I have also discovered some benefits of intermittent fasting and I tell a people during my talks. They are reasons people love my spa too. So, here I will tell you all benefits you sure didn't know about Intermittent fasting.

It's Your Surefire Chance To Keep Your Weight In Your Control

The first reason I will ever recommend Intermittent Fasting to anyone is weight loss. To most people too, the first sign that will mention your Intermittent Fasting to anyone is your weight.

You do not even have to try all methods before you notice that it really helps you shed off your fats. Intermittent Fasting places your weight loss right in your palms. No side effects, no excess. Do whatever you like with it.

You can easily measure your calorie intake, current state and need with an online calculator

I notice, the first fact people discover about fasting is that anyone who has been fasting unconsciously usually lose weight. It is why that your friend who ate only once or twice a day because her family or friend died would look very lean.

Many ladies in the US have realized this fact, and most would skip meals deliberately. Ask the moms, the teenage girls don't eat till you threaten not to buy their lipsticks. My 7-year-old girl promised to jail me if I stuff too much food in her lunch pack, imagine that.

If you are not going to act like you are very innocent yourself, I put it to you that you are reading this book to discover tricks to shed off some weight. Innocent? You can't tell me that, it is written in your eyes and that's why you are still reading me.

Anyway, 100,000 girls are exactly as guilty as you, so feel no sin.

Intermittent Fasting can be the salvation you want on your weight loss actually, and that is why most American mothers, entertainers and even athletes are turning it to the business of the day.

You do not even have to worry about the nature of your food, eat wherever you desire. All you need study is the total calorie, intake, and amount to be lost during Intermittent Fasting.

As long as you have subscribed to any intermittent fasting method, you run the show, and your weight is in trouble!

It's Another Step Away From Cancer

Every single human on earth has got cancer, you know? Cancer is caused by virus and we can be affected in a million ways.

Especially being a woman, you've got breast, ovary, lungs, skin, this, and that cancer, if you still want to be the apple of everyone's eye, you just can't afford to be exposed to it!

Believe it or not, we can all be attacked by various virus that are transferred from the mother to the child during pregnancy, birth and breastfeeding. But most of these viruses don't always attack, that is because we have strong antibodies that fight and control them.

Excess fats, as doctors tag it; obesity, is one of those factors that can weaken the reaction of these antibodies. Bear in mind that once you weaken your defense, your enemies will attack.

Ever played the 'game of city'? you let down your guards and vampire tear down your roof.

So, virus will attack from all angles if you let down your guards.

That's when your mouth and your anus begin to give back what you thought you have digested.

Ever stooled and vomited simultaneously?

That is even simple if you are faced by some almighty viral attacks, let's not talk bulimia.

So, indirectly, you participate in an activity that saves your weight and you're fighting virus!

No doctor would probably tell you this, may be because they are yet to officially confirm how much Intermittent Fasting can help.

But from my three years of practice and co-running a health spa, I can boldly take the bullhorn and shout to the street that Intermittent Fasting is not working on your obesity alone; your inflammation; another primary cause of cancer is in serious battle.

You End Up With A Better Brain And A Better Body

My colleague at the health spa who happened to be a doctor once told me after we saw a Tv show, 'if you have a kid with a poor brain, place him on some periodic Fasting and watch what he eats.' wow.

I wonder, is that not say Intermittent Fasting works for the brain too? Gorgeous.

I planned to confirm it with my baby when she turns 2 years older, but my body attested to it before my baby's.

I doubled as an accountant in another firm when I started my Intermittent Fasting, and part of my worries was that I couldn't keep up with the figures.

They were becoming hard to calculate with my brain and my brain was getting lazier, all I wanted more was sleep. If you have ever been in my shoes, I am sure you will notice every unusual change the moment your brain revolutionizes its working style. I noticed it a few weeks after I started a stable fasting routine. I surprisingly did. I didn't notice at first till it became really clear that something was working on my brain.

I saw my therapist a Sunday after and asked him if there could be some connection with my intermittent fasting. 'a lot' he said, all booming with smiles. 'in a recent research first tried with rats, we discovered that intermittent fasting can increase the ability to learn and use the memory.

Rats on intermittent fast are better protected from many neurological disorders too'. Researches are still on for humans, but they haven't proven contrary so far.

I picked a point from there, Intermittent Fasting is helping the brain. Did anyone ever mention Autophagy to your ears, we are coming to talk about it.

Another confusing secret is that it may weaken your sexual spirit, but it weakens every reason you shouldn't become pregnant too. So, you finding a baby or you trying to weaken your sexual urge? Either ways, go for it.

Among Other Gifts, You Are Awarded a Healthy Heart

'Miss Meg, your cholesterol is on a very dangerous level and it really can be fatal if it moves two inches higher' a doctor complained to me when I stopped by from work one evening.

Three months after, he said to me, 'this is a really remarkable development Ms. Meg, what did you do to yourself?

Your cholesterol really reduced!' I was all smiles that day, and I knew I hadn't done anything, I merely started intermittent fasting.

That was how I got to know too, that apart from brain fitness and carbs control, even my breathing, and my heart is wholesomely affected.

There is a kind of fat in the blood that can cause variety of diseases, they call it Triglycerides. Triglycerides will be present in you if you have too much fats, and that means breathing difficulty, coupled with a bundle of heart diseases.

I have a feeling you don't want me to detail how these things can rotten your heart while you're still walking the street.

But despite all those threats, a consistent cure as simple as intermittent fasting can send them all packing.

I am no physician, but I am going to tell you that my days with top rated doctors, my experience at spa sessions, my interviews with my deeply affected clients and my own studies have established to me that another simple formula to care for cardiovascular functions is Intermittent Fasting.

Isn't it amazing that by simply going on food strike you can save yourself from blood pressure, heart attack, breathing difficulty, and so many others issues, so many solutions, all in one just one pack, intermittent fasting?

Give it to my ears again!

Diabetes? No Way!

As long as you are committed to your fasting routine, one of the attacks you are not likely to have is Type 2 Diabetes.

Type 2 Diabetes is that type of Diabetes that is caused by obesity. I really hate to think about how much fat people are exposed to various diseases. So many problems, and to my complete disgust, diabetes is included!

Three out of every fat lady has a high rate level of glucose and insulin which can lead to diabetes. You are probably one of the three affected. But you need not worry, fasting consistently can help you see off diabetes before it ever rises.

That is why you need to include a stable Intermitting Fasting in your timetable. The only aspect that may cause concern is the assumption that Intermittent Fasting reduces Type 2 Diabetes, not others.

What if it actually increases the others? What if it actually reduces the others too? No research has proven either though, what the records keep proving is that Intermittent Fasting is save, for average humans.

Be The 21st Century Darling

Have you noticed how the modern ladies look stunning? Have you noticed the sexy curves and shapes of most models? Have you discovered that none, I repeat, none of them is fat? You are in the 21st century darling, don't live a 19th century life.

Married or single, tantalizing women now dress in tight fitting dresses, with curvaceous shapes, and fairly slim bodies, nobody is fat. Even the secretaries, and the C.E.O.s and the attendants, and the mother of three and the... you name it! NOBODY IS FAT.

To make things worse, men are now in a crazy hunt for gracefully slender angels that they can wrap up in their hands.

I wonder who put that into their skulls, though wondering who doesn't matter again, all that matters is, they don't want fat girls and you can't afford to be one!

Many husbands get frustrated if they married a gracefully slender curvy girl, but she turned along the line of the relationship to the fattest woman in the street.

Hell, you're making him feel like he's married his grandmother, and men really hate that. Not when curvy girls swam their work place on daily basis.

You don't want health complications, you don't want to be an eyesore at the party, you want to rock shoes and dresses better, you want to look smart and fitting, you want to be everyone's 21st century darling at the first sight? Okay, intermittent fasting, period!

Generally, you will have a very healthy body system if you intermittently fast. You are likely saved from Diabetes, Heart problems, excess sugar, calories, overweight and many other problems too. you will remain the center of attraction everywhere you turn.

Single men, married, gays, even lesbians, all heads must turn your way as you step in the door. Organizations will find it a lot more exciting to have you with them. It's the golden age, and you are the gold.

Chapter 2: Risks Associated to Long Term Fasting

If you think about these benefits, you won't even want to assume Intermittent Fasting has dark sides, but yes, it's got a bunch of really grievous ones. Before you try anything, I suggest you go through these risks associated to long term Intermittent Fasting and measure the statistics.

Are you fit for the game? Right now, I'm talking about fasting for as long as 6 months to 2 years.

There are just a handful of them problems.

Though, all too important to be left unmentioned because they can determine your health and safety too.

Really, really awful things.

Hunger Can Threaten Your Senses

Do you know hunger?

Have you really experienced hunger before?

I'm not talking about those few times you return from work, famished and exhausted. I'm talking real churning anger that could make one man seem seven to your face. I mean the kind of hunger that would make the girl in your mirror look like your grandmother.

To be frank with you, when you are on Intermittent Fasting, sometimes you don't eat anything for as long as 16 hours in a day, sometimes 20 of 24 hours.

Do you have any idea how you could feel at lunch break when the last time you had a meal was dinner last night and none was in view until supper?

Ever been so hungry you can't see what the computer writes. The letters keep popping up together and mixing into each other in your eyes, you can't hold a thing, you can't stand on your feet without shivering and all you really want to do is eat.

It doesn't get any easier if you are on the 5/2 diet where you are banned from half your foods and even roughages for two solid days.

Have you ever been in the shoes of someone who had no meals and had no choice but to go to bed? You can imagine how they spend their nights counting the window sills and rolling about the bed?

I hate to tell you that hunger is one of the agents that can make your sense organs malfunction, and Intermittent Fasting can invite you some master class hunger.

Hunger can cause you to feel weak, tired, not to think straight and to awfully go about your business of the day.

Apart from feeling nasty and unhealthy, you are probably exposed to stomach ache, head ache, cancer, ulcer and some other bad 'cers' again, isn't that bad enough? You don't dare hunger, you just don't. And trying intermittent fasting, especially for a long period of time means hunger.

For me however, I felt my hunger just at the start, my body surprisingly got really well along, I didn't feel pangs and I didn't want to eat my colleagues out of hunger, I just got along really well. Worked for me, there are just chances it could for you too. Chances.

You Can Become Quick Tempered Forever

One of my fear for people who engage in Intermittent Fasting for a long period is that they can lose their sense of humor.

You know how they say it? Happiness is from within, and a woman who is really hungry is likely to be angry. If you happen to fast at some time of the week, work with a couple of zany bosses who slam any one and couple this with a late month menstrual pain, I bet you are likely to be the maddest woman in America.

Nobody is happy when they are angry, are you?

Your hunger is enough a cause of pain and anger, and you probably could have managed the other issues better without hunger.

Now, nobody dares cross your lane because that will mean they are daring a hungry leopard. You would begin to get angry at anyone and everyone. Not exactly your fault, just the result of the battles and protests raised in your belly by some idiotic hungry enzymes.

This is one bad effect Long period of fasting can have on any lady.

If you don't want to slam into your client's face because he's pricing your goods too low, you don't want to slap the kid just for spilling some milk, you don't want to end up hating everyone who eats right in front of you, you don't want to become this irritable person that would never feel free to dance and rock the dance floor because you're hungry. you don't want to lose your patience over these rigmaroles you've always done at work suddenly, I really am afraid you must not for any reason take up intermittent Fasting for a long period of time.

Less, you unconsciously find yourself meeting all of the above qualifications.

You know what being an asshole means to your boyfriend?

Mom will never call too, clients will never stop by your desk, your kids will prefer their dad and if you are single, hell, boys, will prefer your maid to you. So, if the goal is still to look smart and not irritable, Intermittent Fasting must not be continued for long.

Weakness

Our studies show that at least 15% more of women practicing now are really interested in Intermittent Fasting. Trouble is they don't want look dull and weak at work like a beaten waterleaf.

You know how horrible it is when everyone keeps asking you why you look so dull and weak at work.

Yeah, if Intermittent Fasting was sued to court on the count of making people feel weak, I agree it will be found guilty without exoneration.

I don't want to scare you, but if you an athlete and you think you have the strength, the zeal and the spirit to fast for six months and still lead the games, I am predicting that fasting will sap you in full.

Fasting for long is not ideal for athletes.

Usually, you would expect yourself to feel lighter and perhaps have the strength to move from one place to another, you will enjoy it if you are an athlete or swimmer or something along those lines, but nobody should do it for long.

Athletes are even likely to enjoy the spirit of a lighter body and a faster brain and spirit, but don't hope to continue the chain.

Just don't continue the cycle. Going on for long can make you so light that with just a push, you are off the floor.

Just imagine, you find yourself on the street, a crazy car whizzes by while chasing another, just the wind hits you and your legs sway you off the floor.

Or let's suppose you are in a busy market and a couple of boys who owe each other something ran by you, pushed you lightly and bash! You crashed.

How do you explain what made you so light to the people around? I really hate embarrassments and I tell you, you have invited more of it once you find yourself on a queue at the bank, on a mad Monday rush or a night crowd pushing one another, you become everyone's pushover since you are really weak and tired. Going on a long fasting spree can also cut your weight than you desire. Everyone is just going to keep asking you at work, 'Holy christ Gray, you look like hell!'.

Weakness gets to its peak psychologically, physically, sexually, morally, motivationally, and every ally you can think of. You just won't be able to explain what happened to yourself.

Your boyfriend is tired because you can't take him hard in bed anymore. Your Boss, your Dad, your friends, everyone is saying you aren't what you used to be, even you are tired of everything. All for just one reason, you fasted too long and became too weak!

You May Be Exposed To Health Dangers Again

Why did you want to pick up Intermittent Fasting? To keep a healthy and fit and smart body right?

I know, but how does it feel to think that this same intermittent fasting that cures and prevents a hundred of problem can also cause a hundred more if continued over a long period of time? Ouch, I hate to think about that side actually, but we need to talk about it.

Remember I told you Intermittent Fasting can save you from Type 2 Diabetes, have you wondered, 'what happened to the other types?'

It's not proven, but as long as nobody is sure, you may be exposed to other types of diabetes especially if you continue for a long period of time.

That is even simple, what if you find yourself embattling ulcer merely because you want to keep a healthy and smart look? You got some kind of serious problems because you want to solve some kind of other problems. Seriously, how sonorous is that?

Nobody has fully confirmed that Intermittent Fasting is a direct cause of ulcer, but if you continue to stab your lungs and bellies and kidneys for a long period of time, what happens?

Fasting Intermittently for a long period, as a year of more can even mean more danger.

Let's not even link it with menstruation, pregnancy and some core female's complications for now. It can make you just lose interest in food without explanation.

Your doctors might begin to say you are losing excess salt and water. You should notice that your skin looks three years older than your old skin. You may suffer from loss of sleep among so many other problems.

Those figures aren't really nice, and they worry the doctors too.

That's probably why they are thinking twice before they recommend it. It is even important to mention, your body may not be happy to welcome the sort of changes that fasting for a long period of time can cause, and that's why you still need to talk to a doctor before trying it.

Intermittent fasting is in many ways better than most other types of fasting, especially those religions like Islam and Christianity engage in, but not ever, you heard that right, not ever should you even plan of trying it for a long period of time.

Your Body May Change, Not In A Good Way

So many things have to stop if you fast for a long period of time. Sometimes, because you feel too weak to continue, you lost the vibe or fasting no longer permits that.

For me, I don't think it's beautiful to stop playing my Sunday squash or lacrosse or my baking classes or calisthenics ({giggles}men love fits girls), and so many others because I am on some mission for a healthy body.

All these helps build a healthy body too and I might have to stop them because I don't have the strength to continue? No way.

Have you seen any other version of yourself?

I mean have you seen a 'you' who hates what you would like, a 'you' who wouldn't eat what you would lick the plates over, a complicated 'you' in a refined you? I bet you haven't, and you don't want to. You don't want the 'you' that hates your old sleeping schedule, your dietary table, your cycle of friends, your pool of parties and even your favorite colors, everything the awkward 'you' want is the opposite of what you would!

I for one don't want that, and I didn't get that anyway. But that's because I didn't try Intermittent Fasting for such a long period as a year.

If you plan to fast that long, then you should get ready to change your system, because your body may not react the way it used to any longer.

Let's take it this way, a lady who's on a 20/4 intermittent fasting for as long as a year for instance, would have missed some scintillating meals she used to enjoy.

Your favorite morning beacons, the mashed potatoes, mid-morning sandwich and so many others you used to love but couldn't take because you have only 4 hours to eat each day and you can't cram all your favorites into such a brief period. By the time that year ends, you just realize you no longer love those things. Are you planning a different you?

So it is important that you know, a lot of not-too-good changes can occur because you're Fasting, especially if you're doing it for a long period of time.

There's not a thing on mother planet that doesn't has its bad sides you know. Intermittent Fasting is worth your efforts, go back and see the advantages again.

But you might really be saving yourself a bunch of complications if you keep it moderate, not for a long period and not that brief if you want to feel the effects.

So, are we planning intermittent fasting for a long period of time?

Cheers, we both know the answer.

Chapter 3: Autophagy and Intermittent Fasting

Who else uses a brain that doesn't process anything the first time they hear Autophagy from anyone?

Who cares, I still don't feel guilty about that word, it is built for the hospital and I am not their fan. Auto is the only thing my brain picked the first time and I was sure it means 'self' or to do something by oneself, phagy can stand by the doorway.

But I picked more interest in the word after a doctor mentioned it in one of our sessions. I realize it's one of the mesmerizing gifts that come with intermittent fasting.

Autophagy is a magic that happens inside our body. It's basically about how our body kills itself and resurrects.

Confused? Oh, just come with me! You see, many things happen right inside our body, and we don't even have any idea. It's like our body is a company on its own, the brain and the nervous systems are the board of directors, there are different systems that act like departments to ensure everything flows smoothly.

That's why we have the digestive system, excretory system, reproductive system, endocrine system, nervous system and a host of other systems.

It's just the same way every company would have the finance department, the public relations department, the marketing department, production and what else? I'd better leave that to you. How many more do you remember?

Okay, you should also notice that apart from this classification, each of these branches is also broken into sections.

Let's say the production department in a flour mill is an example, then there's the mixing unit, the grinding unit, the heating unit, and each of these units contain offices too. There's the supervisor, there's the unskilled labor who're found in almost all units and blah blah blah. Is that the same way your company is structured, where do you belong?

You know where it gets interesting, these systems in our body function in that same order. The digestive system for instance includes the mouth, the trachea, the small intestines and every other organ that has something to do in digestion. In their own case, the unskilled labors in our body systems are called cells.

There are billions of cells in the human body, very tiny things. You can see them in every living thing, even plants. You can think of them the same way you see the unskilled workers who actually do most of the real works in the company.

You know how biologists define them? 'the basic unit of life'. Oh hell, I think I sound like a biologist myself, but even if biology is interesting, I can't stand the terminologies.

I know you want to ask me what cells have got to do with intermittent fasting, and you're already asking yourself since you can't see me. Just relax okay? You'll find the nexus soon.

The first thing you'll remember about unskilled workers is that they are strong, they don't work for long and usually they don't live long.

Sometimes, they are changed to another position, sometimes, they die, they leave work, they are fired when they get old and all of those things that can happen to them.

That's exactly what the cells in our body do too, but rather than leave work, they commit suicide. Funny isn't it?

I don't think our brain and other directors are capitalists, so they aren't overusing the cells, it's just the cells often realize they can't do much for the company any longer and what do they do? Suicide.

They die but they are magically reused in that stunning manner that, they give birth to newer, younger and much more vibrant cells. That's only in a standard temperature and pressure.

You know what I mean? In a standard situation where you supply your body the required nutrients regularly, that's what happens. And that process is exactly what they call **Autophagy**.

So Autophagy, in a lay-man sense, is the process by which old cells in our body murder themselves and are reused to form younger, livelier, stronger and better cells.

So, is autophagy still strange? I don't think it should be strange anymore, I think it should be funny.

But for autophagy to happen, there's got to be some situations in place. First, you are feeding your body all the nutrients it needs in the proper proportion.

Then, you allow the body enough space to carry out autophagy. How? If you keep stuffing your belly with food and anything that comes near your mouth, the way a fish stuffed herself with everything including Jonah, God's apostle, you aren't giving autophagy a chance.

All you're doing is eating and giving the body enough strength to produce new set of cells without disturbing the old ones.

The old ones get too tired, too weak and constitute mere nuisance to the body, when in fact they could have been used to produce other cells. That's why you would notice that your skin is rough sometimes, your digestion is slow, you are weak despite eating and so forth.

You have a strange mix up of workers! Once these confusion gets too extreme, the young and old will all grow old and refuse to be used, new ones will be formed and your organs will be so choked that you would look old, ugly and possibly die for it.

You don't even have to overstuff your belly like Jonah's captor before this happens, it would happen if you use a three square meal all day of the week. Remember there are fruits and drinks and mid-morning brunt too.

Now, the easiest way out of this? Intermittent Fasting! Can you please say that to my ears again? Very good!

If you fast intermittently, you have given your body system a chance at autophagy which means you will likely have a fresher skin, look younger and more likely live longer. If you don't want that, show me your hand. You didn't raise your hand.

Then, let's talk about the class of people who can fast and those who really shouldn't.

Who should fast?

As it happens, you don't need to be tangled in a problem before you have it all solved. So, even if you don't have real excess fats to burn, intermittent fasting is a good way to maintain your weight.

I advise young ladies to try intermittent fasting. That's because it's a safe trick from sexual, marital and birth complications. It keeps your skin radiant, as I've told you while explaining autophagy. I guess holy spirit already spoke to the high schoolers, they somehow made sure they never complete their diet. Ask the moms.

Married women and those with kids should try intermittent fasting too.

Especially those who notice that their bellies continue to bulge like a balloon even after giving birth. Nothing is wrong with you medically, but your man married a flat portable lady, not a balloon bellied.

He may love you a lot alright, but don't give him a chance to think about other women he meets every day at work who have what you used to have.

I'm still going to discuss the chances of working women and intermittent fasting in full, just a few pages away.

So if you ask me, intermittent fasting is for all girls, ladies, women. As long as there's no health complication of any sort initially.

Who shouldn't fast?

Now what happens if you have a couple of health problems before?

I hate to tell you that it really may not be a brilliant idea to try out intermittent fasting. Although, the complexity determines your chances of trying intermittent fasting.

For instance, if it's some menstrual pain that stops with menstruations, and your monthly flow doesn't flow like you are a planning to fill a tank, you shouldn't have a problem trying intermittent fasting.

But you might face real issues if you usually have overflow of blood and you fast again.

If you are underweight, or you have been told that rather than lose some, you need more weight, I would cross out any chance of fasting if I were you.

If you are usually anxious too or your doctors are still trying to get you working on a healthy feeding style, the numerous benefits may be too attractive to leave, but your weight and focus must be on your body balance.

Some people think it's a bad idea to let kids fast. Well, a young woman who hasn't started her menses may try intermittent fasting, just that there are chances her puberty could be delayed if she fasted for too long.

So, it's always advised that when your little chubby girl tries it, it is once in a while. Just once a few times and she'll be safe.

Apart from such kind of problems, if you are on a constant diet of some kind, or perhaps drugs and you might have to pause them to fast, it makes no sense to even hope to.

If you are a cancer, ulcer or one of the few other 'cers' patient, I think it makes sense to see your doctor before starting any diet plan.

Apart from these few conditions, we also need to talk about a couple other states, everyone can fast, except some I want to mention below.

A Woman On Menstruation.

As I guess you would be aware, that monthly blood that breaks from a woman's vagina and flows at regular times is called menstruation.

We know it goes on for a few days, sometimes 3, and 8 at most. Does yours go longer than that?

That means you have to see a doctor urgently, before you even think of a diet table.

If yours is okay, then 'we can probably calculate your chances of fasting intermittently together', as Dr. Roberts would say.

Because menstruation can make you feel weak, you need your strength, your stamina, your meals and all calories you can get during your monthly flow.

But fasting means your body gets only a few supplies.

If you are not planning a very long intermittent fasting period, and you live a very healthy life before, you shouldn't have any problem with fasting because there's this nutrient reserve inside you that your body turns to for help.

If that's not the case, intermittent fasting could mean that the part of your brain that coordinate your regular monthly flow called 'hypothalamus' will be too hungry to work, and gonadotropin releasing hormones (those ones see to your monthly flow in the ovaries) and the pituitary gland are affected too. what happens? You bag irregular and disrupted menstrual cycle.

It can even get worse if you are on a long period intermittent fasting because your nutrient reserve will likely be too low to supply enough calories, and it can get to that point where your body system switches off your reproductive organs.

It says "hey, close that baby factory, this girl has got nothing to feed a baby, so just shut the doors, we open when she has enough nutrients to fund our business again'.

Of course, you can have sex but the eggs won't be formed. The moment you supply enough nutrients, that body system returns to normal.

So, on mensuration, should you fast during intermittent fasting? Tell me, I'm all ears.

Pregnancy

Dear potbellied sister, I am going to be very frank with you right now.

You love something doesn't make it ideal for you. Intermittent fasting can really help your brain, burn your fats, help your cells reproduction and help your food digestion, yes, I know all of them.

But I am sorry to tell you, your pregnancy ends your fast, till delivery at least.

Why? Because you've got a baby inside your stomach who doesn't bloody care about all those hellacious treatments you are finding yourself.

It needs you to have more weight, meaning more fats, more sugar and to eat any possible thing at any time they come like the biblical fish that ate everything, including Jonah.

So, fasting for a pregnant? Possible, just not ideal.

Breast-feeding

Now let's turn to the baby mothers.

Hey bouncing baby mother! How are you? Has your ballooned belly refused to deflate after delivery? Have you tripled your size despite delivery and now you want me to tip you?

Forget the jokes, you are asking the right person.

It's okay to still have a very large tummy after birth. Or a kind of weight around that old size you had while pregnant.

It is okay, but if you can return to the former gracefully slender lady that everyone knew, why hold on to an old version?

Dr. Macron had often repeated that breast feeding women can practice intermittent fasting too. Most women were always fat in his own home after delivery.

So they mildly practiced intermittent fasting after delivery and they were fine. So, dear mother, it's a yes.

But I have to ring in it your head as we were taught, you need about 1800 calories to supply nutritious milk per day, how do you plan to supply that for over a year if you are not getting it yourself?

Well, if you are keeping it as mild as possible, say only 8-10 hours per day. That's on a 10:14 fasting to eating ratio. You are not likely to be affected, and you can gradually tackle all inflammation, you can even ensure autophagy that way.

So, if you must fast, strictly make it no longer than I said.

A Woman On Menopause

Hi granny! We got your package too. While it is very possible to reach menopause (that's when you don't menstruate anymore) at 47, the ideal age is about 58 upwards.

Your autophagy rate will likely reduce as you grow older, but becoming a grandma doesn't mean you have to suffer from excess insulin, calories fat, a dull brain, an unhealthy digestive system and inflammation among others right?

Great, I really think you should try intermittent fasting.

There was this old and very grey haired woman among us who was always complaining because she was too fat and her legs would not take her oversized body anywhere.

I know she got a lot better after fasting, but she probably did it for a very long period which I don't recommend for old women. Short periods can cure you too.

Intermittent fasting can boost your immunity, your digestion, your brain functioning, your balance weight campaign and of course your general healthiness.

It's worth a trial really, but be careful, I don't want to be told you fasted for forty days, you are already too old to be Jesus.

So if you are among those I said can practice intermittent fasting, then be sure you do it moderately, don't toy with a baby's neural growth just because you want less fat, make it moderate.

But as people often ask me, if you are a very busy woman, does it make sense to try intermittent fasting?

Chapter 4: Intermittent Fasting For A Busy Woman

Who wants to be a sleep-at-home wife these days?

I know some of those second and third world countries are still engaging in that, but not here in America, not here. Right now, I am beginning to wonder if women don't work than men.

As a first world woman, you find yourself in an extremely hectic schedule.

You spend the best parts of the day filing papers, drafting letters, attending to clients, battling death for a client's life, finding facts on a dirty politician and so many other assignments.

Depending on your job. But somehow, you still managed to gather so many fats that you know you are standing in the yellow zone, you continue that way and you enter the red zone.

Should you fast too? As Dr Robert's would say, 'let's calculate your chances of intermittent fasting together'.

First, how busy are you? Are you among the first few drivers every morning and you're always among the last on the street at night, that is if you aren't flying to Houston right from office. Or are you the store keeper who opens the store at 9 and closes by 4pm? Yours might even be tighter.

We need to earmark one fact at the start of our analysis; you are going to need a lot of energy for your daily tasks.

Running up and down streets, sitting and standing, going and coming all require a chunk of energy, which is usually generated from the calories, carbs and fats you consume.

Now if you are boycott that food, how does your body get energy? You can't even hope to rely on your body reserve, because people who are too busy don't usually have enough calories in their reserve, so don't think about it.

A Tv show in Bosnia Herzegovina just confirmed that most very busy women interviewed on the show often miss most of them meals.

They forget to order, sometimes order and forget to eat. To me, they are already practicing intermittent fasting. I can imagine what it feels like. you leave home hoping to catch breakfast at a fast spot, end up thinking it's going to be late so get to work with nothing in your stomach.

Even the few times you stopped by or ordered for it, only 3% is eaten, you get too busy to smell the rest. The cycle goes for breakfast and lunch and even dinner. All you have in your stomach is drink and fast snacks.

A similar research conducted by a European women health magazine reveals that most busy women follow the healthy eating formula.

That is the principle that you should feed on fruits twice and normal foods three times a day. You haven't started intermittent fasting, but tell me, how many of these diets do you take religiously? That's the point.

Don't look at me like you're innocent, we both know you skip them.

But despite skipping them, you still happen to be overweight, or let's say because of the various other benefits, you are really interested in Intermittent Fasting. Not a bad idea, I think.

Intermittent Fasting can at least prevent excess fats from storing, so, let's draft a plan for you.

Take a calculator and begin to note, how many hours are you going off-diet already? Can you afford three, five more hours without meal and you won't hear lousy noises that can kill your spirit from your stomach? Your work is important, but if you can keep fit and healthy, it's a lot more important.

You may go a variety of diet plans, maybe just open your eating window for 8-10 hours.

Most times, I advise you fix your intermittent fasting during your busiest hours, since you won't have the time to eat anyway.

All you need take is a cup of green tea, Oolong Tea or perhaps coffee. Any liquid that suits you. But less of alcohol. Remember the tank in your belly is empty, you don't want to fill it with acidic drinks that can spur cancer. you're on a 16:8 for instance. You can fast from 9pm- 1pm the next day.

All you boycotted was breakfast and that's not new anyway, it only has to be more regular now and no kitchen business in the midnight. There are many other plans, and I'll tell you about them soon.

Intermittent Fasting And Sport

Ladies who engage in sport are among the healthiest ladies I know.

They watch the amount of calories they consume on daily basis, they watch their sleep, their wears and even drinks. But this freestyle weight control strategy called Intermittent Fasting is attracting interest so much that they want to know if it works for them too.

Like it would be on yours if you were a sportswoman, the first thing on the question of most sportswomen is if they can try intermittent fasting without weakening their performance.

No doubt, you need to be sure you'd still make the first team and you still display their magnificent talents without dropping form.

But up till this moment, there hasn't been a standard research on how much Intermittent fasting can affect an athlete's career. What a French medic corporation, the closest researcher on this case reports is that

Athletes are likely affected by Intermittent Fasting negatively.

Athletes calorie intake determines the amount of energy they can expend on the lines. So, if you reduce your calorie intake, your energy likely reduces.

Roffeinham, an African-American medical researcher based in Ukraine also thinks you might feel very light and probably weak.

If you continue fasting for a long time too, you can even blackout in a game.

These researches concluded with something however, if your body needs to shed some weight to look smarter and fitter for the game.

Go for Intermittent Fasting, it'll increase your tolerance, endurance and of course your fitness.

I am no sport colossus, but I really believe you can try intermittent fasting too. You need a fast and light brain and body, a body that can endure too.

Since Intermittent Fasting can give you that, a 16:8 might be your best shot too.

Chapter 5: Types Of Intermittent Fasting

Before we go further, remember Intermittent Fasting is just a deliberate act of shying away from food some specific time after which you eat again.

Most times when you meet people who own health spas, we like to classify Intermittent Fasting to only two.

So every other classification is hidden inside them.

The easy type of Intermittent Fasting

That's what we call the simplest methods if Intermittent Fasting.

Just before you call for my head, I know they may not be that simple for everyone, and they look typically difficult for starters, I agree. But if you compare them with some other methods, yes.

You'll agree that each of them is a piece of cake. Which of them are you familiar with?

a. The Time Window Game: This is an absolute game of time. You keep timing yourself every day. What time is it, when do I start, and when do I end? Usually, you split your 24 hours into fasting hours and eating hours. You can begin this by cutting two hours before your dinner and increasing breakfast time by an hour and ensuring you eat nothing after dinner till the next time you're eating hours begin. Let's assume you have your dinner by 9pm and breakfast by 8 in the morning and yes, no snacks, no fruits till the next 8am after dinner. You can shrink this to 7pm at night and 9 in the morning. It is later reduced to 10am-6pm, till you feel open to more adjustments. You only have to make it regular, or perhaps increase but not decrease it. Some common ones are;

> 14/10 fasting window; here, the plan is that you go on a vibrant and empty belly for 14 of 24 hours every day. Most of these hours are lost in the night when you don't eat anyway, so this is going to be very easy for you. You only have to steer off midnight crunches. You can also o weave it around your busiest hours. This should work well if you merely want to practice for overweight prevention.

> 16/8 fasting window; the 16/8 is merely an improvement on the 14/10 fasting method. Add two more hours to your fast and feel more effects. You may even begin with this method. That's what I tell breastfeeding mothers or single ladies who are worried about their monthly flow. Our records prove that this and the other above do not usually affect menstruation.

b. The weekend or 5/2 fasting window; another easy one where you eat all of your normal diets every single day, but you cut them drastically in two days every week. That doesn't have to be weekends, I suggest your busiest days of the week. This method says you can go on with 3 sumptuous meals every day for 5 days and gain about 1200 calories on daily basis (this varies a lot), you only have to cut the calorie intake to no more than 350-450 in two days. It is possible really.

Just tell your body there's little food in the next two days, it will understand, it always.

That will keep your weight in check for real. Our bodies have an amazing way of adjusting, so yours will no doubt listen to you too.

You are not staying off meals, just reducing them. Most of you skip many meals anyway, so it will be no big deal. This works better for ladies who engage in sports.

The Hard Types of Intermittent Fasting

Hey, I caught you! You read that again. Why? Oh come on. Just as the simple type isn't as simple as it sounds, this isn't as difficult as it sounds too. It is meant for strong women.

It is a challenge every woman above 210 pounds should take. You just tell yourself it is simple and it is done too. There are two known types:

a. The alternative Fasting: don't be deceived by the name, we didn't make fasting an alternative for you overweights. We mandate it. It's just you alternate your fasting periods. You fast today and take practically all of your diets again tomorrow. Sometimes you can take half or nothing at all on fasting days. For instance, you can have your sumptuous calories as usual, that's around 1,200 calories (varies according to body needs). The next day, you should have half or less throughout the day. Sometimes, fast on 0 calories. Hard? Maybe, but yes. You can. Any woman above 150 is fat so, she can afford it. You may however stop by your doctor's to get suggestions. Do you get it? Read it again.

b. The Eat: Stop: Eat method; this method gave itself away from its name. It's about eating for a while, stopping, eating for a while again and the cycle circles. Don't get too excited, that 'while' isn't hours, it is days. So, you eat for a few days, fast for a day or two (that's 24-48 donkey hours) resume eating again. I used this actually. I would rotate my fasting period. Sometimes, once a week, sometimes twice. it's very fast, yeah, I'll tell you that, and effective. But don't go on for long, it's not a very thrilling experience to sit at a party all day and keep your gut shut, or travel all-round the city on a rampaging stomach.

As far as the records point, these are the most common, notable and most used structures of Intermittent Fasting.

You may come up with a different and more convenient pattern of course, but it may be difficult to measure your progress in comparison with other people who are fasting intermittently. So!

Where do you fall, what's your choice? Shall we talk about how you can start now?

Chapter 6: How to get started as beginners

Starting Intermittent Fasting is like getting home after listening to a thorough sermon at church.

You tell yourself 'no more am I doing this. No more am I doing that' and so on.

If you talk straight to your soul, you can actually change from that moment. Just in that same spirit, you need some tête-a-tête with your mind, so you won't end up cheating after 3 days.

On another hand, there are chances you won't get frustrated to the point of cheating if it is simple enough, so it really ought to be, that's right. Because of that, I have compiled a couple of simple tips that can guarantee you a thrilling experience.

I will also tell you the best things you should put into your mouth when fasting and what you should not go near, just right under this.

Simple precautions to start fasting

1. Determine your objectives; what's the target? What exactly do you want to achieve? That should help you determine how long and how far your fasting should go. Is this a precaution against overweight or a cure, is it for autophagy or just healthiness? You need to consider your safety and your calorie needs before deciding. As a case study, I started out with a determination to lose 220 of 310 pounds. The report? I did in 7 months on a eat-stop-eat diet.

2. Consider what your nature supports: what does your nature allows? A cancer patient won't find it thrilling to go on a 20: 4 diet, neither would a breast feeding or pregnant one. A busy woman can afford this however. So, confirm your needs and your daily life before deciding too, lest you become a regular, not at the health spa but the hospital.

By your estimate. Which of the plans will you start with? How long? A year?

What are the best things you can eat?

You are open to a very wide range of alternative of dietary contents during intermittent fasting. I really am glad to remind you that this isn't marathon fasting, and it's not Ramadan.

So, the kind of constrictions Christians and Muslims place on their fast may not exactly apply here. We all know none of them would allow eating or drinking that period of fasting. But intermittent fasting allows drinking especially, eating is banned too.

That's because what you are fasting for your body to sue up the excess calories and supplying it with other calories during the fasting can't make that happen.

You can take water of any kind, hot, ice, warm or bottled, take mint tea, red tea, ginger, chamomile and if the last option, coffee, but nonalcoholic drinks should be taken really lightly, remember they are filled to the brim with sugar, in essence, calories which you are staying away from at that period.

I always recommend no intake of alcohol because it could cause burns in your organs. It works like very hot and acidic liquids poured into a shiny but empty tank.

In the image that comes to your mind, you'll realize that such tanks can rust too easily.

Sure enough You don't want to say hi to kidney, lungs and their sister cancers and you don't want to damage your internal system.

When your fasting window closes and the dining spring comes, eat any eatable entity that suits your taste. Anything. As long as you want it.

Though, it tops my recommendation that you eat foods that have high calorie content, or at least make them appear regularly in your diet timetable. That means they can supply you enough calories to energize your day and you won't feel deep effects of fasting.

An average human needs 800-1400 calories a day. But you may need more especially during your menstrual cycle.

What shouldn't eat during intermittent fasting

There are a couple of things that you shouldn't dare during Intermittent Fasting.

The top of them, no pizzas, potatoes, hamburgers, no real foods during your fasting window. Anything that can supply your body with sugar or calories should be avoided.

Your nonalcoholic drinks aren't innocent in this case too.

Chewing gums, lolly. Every single one of them has got sugar. What's the point in fasting when you still keep supplying your body what you're asking it to throw away? Just the drinks I mentioned earlier would suffice.

No drugs, no exotic alcohols too. I tried alcohol once and nobody, not even the boss who fired me for no reason will try it before my eyes, that stomach churn

I got was the standard definition of agony.

When your eating window opens? Wine and dine in your vineyard as you desire. But as I mentioned earlier, take more of things that can boost your calories.

Your stomach no doubt feels awkward and light, don't overstuff it or you end up pouring out the rest from your mouth and nostrils.

Chapter 7: Common Mistakes To Avoid During Intermittent Fasting.

Now that you have trapped all the secrets behind Intermittent Fasting in your palms, I bet you can't wait to start. I felt that way too.

Why wait? No reason of course. But I should probably spend this moment hinting you that despite fasting intermittently, you may end up not getting your desired result.

Because intermittent Fasting failed? No way. It's because you made some under-the-shoes mistakes. All those petty mistakes nobody takes serious.

I am going to tell you those mistakes most people make, and end up returning to me in confusion.

Some are not very common but you are prone to them too.

You can thank me later, I got them all here.

Choosing a wrong plan

If your body needs a high level of fats, then you shouldn't opt for the hard types of intermittent fasting.

Most people want to see the magic happen so they often opt for the hard ones. Falling on the bad side, they end up with abdominal twinges.

According to *New Times Observation*, those who really need to shed a huge wrap of weight also prefer to go for simple intermittent fasting.

They prefer simple plans that won't cost them drastic cuts in their food intake. It's like taking a medication for kids at 33.

I want to know my fat darling, how does that work?

It is the first reason you should soup the scales, see how much there is to be lost and select what works best for you.

Alternating Methods Out Of Impatience

Right in the words of Krista Varady, PhD, associate professor of kinesiology and nutrition at the University of Illinois, "Some people quit if they start out by fasting for too many hours without an adjustment period from a previous eating style".

You really don't have to frustrate yourself, give it time. Remember you didn't pile your excess fats in one month, don't expect a magical turnaround.

Your body will adjust; it is built for that sort of thing.

Giving Up

Craine Greene, a social psychologist believes that our body has the ability to withstand anything.

After you have exposed it to something different from what it knew for about 30 days, it automatically adjusts.

So, if your head hurts, or your stomach churns, or your belly slams like thunder the first few times you begin, it really is okay.

Your body will adjust and you'll be perfect again with time. Giving up is a ghastly mistake.

Not Waiting For The Results

15 of every woman fasting Intermittently report that they thought they picked the wrong method and flipped to another the first few times they started.

But when they hear the other 5 give witness on these same methods, they knew they should have waited further.

You can cause your body hormonal and psychological imbalance if you continue flipping without stability, or giving up, starting again and repeating that sort of cycle.

Remember your body is a very organized system, it needs to understand you and what exactly your choices are. Stay calm, the results will come.

Overeating

I said you can eat anything remember? But no, I didn't say you should stuff your belly with everything.

Eat the average meal that can supply you the best of nutrients.

You need healthy diets that are especially rich in Protein and Fibers during your fasting periods.

Carbs are important too, you need some regular calorie supply, even if smaller than usual.

I'll list those foods that do the magic in the next chapter.

Not Being Choosy About What You Eat

Yes, we all agreed we can eat anything, but isn't it best to eat the best? Don't eat scavenges, I am not training a scavenger.

Eat the healthiest diets.

I am listing them for you already.

No excuses.

Cheating

Cheating is not always a bad idea during Intermittent Fasting.

Do it just once in a very long while.

You keep cheating and you keep slowing down your own progress.

You should not extend your period of eating beyond the agreed deadline too.

Chapter 8: Permanent Weight Loss Tips.

Permanent Weight Loss

Right now, with a couple of committed intermittent fasting, nobody needs much to dispose of excess fats again. But a fact we have taken time to discuss together is that Intermittent Fasting should not go for long.

It should continue for no more than 6-7 months. After those months. How should you lose weight?

There are a couple of things that you can do and you would lose your weights permanently. I bet you're already thinking they are harder than intermittent fasting, aren't you?

Don't ask for my head yet, I still think they are simpler. Maybe you would too. They are more of habits too. No big rules. You just need to do as many of these as you can:

1. Regular Exercise: Be a sportswoman. It keeps you alive. It keeps your vein and muscles vibrant. It aids

Autophagy too. Remember what that is? Excess salts, fats and sugar are lost every time you excite your spirit with not-so-tedious and deliberate games, like playing on a pedometer. Nobody is asking you to drag a truck. Just Calisthenics. Regularly.

2. More Snacks, less diets: I know that story circulating the house that you eat a mountain of food every time you want to eat isn't exactly true. But I advise, if you want to lose your weights permanently, you have to reduce them. You need to eat less solids and fats, feed more on snacks. Light snacks with high fiber value. Having them a couple of times every day or more, sometimes in place of one of your actual diets can do the magic. Don't spend a day without exercise. Take a walk, jump, stroll to friends. Run out to the fourth street in the morning and make sure you get a long exercise after sitting at a computer for hours.

3. Make sure you read the labels: Many people are especially fond of skipping the instructions and labels on their processed foods, which are not the best anyway. Read them, consider the contents. In the

words of Dr Roger, High Calorie, high sugar, carbs, fats can never help a stable weight loss, avoid them.

4. More fibers, more Protein: Proteins and fibers are what you need to take in most. The Carbs will always crouch in anyway. So look out for foods with that are especially rich in protein, fiber and mild fats.

Are they as difficult as Intermitted Fasting?

May be no, but they are for permanent maintenance, not drastic cut. So.

Don't even hope to replace Intermittent Fasting with them.

KETO DIET

You probably have seen Keto diet in the ads, or on the TV.

Let me tell you a bit about that too. Keto diet is a way of planning your diets so excess carbs would you be scrapped in them, and instead, you have diets with higher fats content.

That can cut down the sugar and insulin levels in your body. You are not likely affected by a ton of diseases. Such diet drives your body to a metabolic state called Ketones.

What's the use? Your body can easily burn most of its fats for energy. So, rather than be fat loaded, you are energy filled.

Variety of Ketogenic or Keto diets are common in town. But what everyone uses is the High Protein Ketogenic diet and Standard Ketogenic diets. The two others; the targeted and cyclic ketogenic diets are for athletes.

The Standard Ketogenic Diet structure your food diet such that 60% of your diet is fat and that'll be converted to energy, 5% is carb and all of the rest is protein.

The standard Ketogenic picks a very percentage of fats too, less protein and lesser carbs. It is very common and most of your diets can be woven around it.

With the scintillating advantages that come with Ketogenic diet, I think it's worth a trial too. For instance;

1. It can help reduce weight.

2. It can break the excess fats no use custom.

3. It does a terrific job against diabetes.

4. Like a sister to Intermittent Fasting, it fights cancers too.

5. It aids your heart, kidney and lungs.

6. According to OAU's Health Sciences Faculty annual publication too, epilepsy Parkinson's disease, brain injuries are areas Ketogenic Diets can give you a hand in.

Now Ketogenic diet Vs Intermittent Fasting?

You know them pretty well now. Ketogenic Diet constricts and most times changes what you eat.

That's something that doesn't interest Intermittent Fasting. The Fast thing doesn't excite people on Keto diets too.

You can practice Ketogenic Diets on Intermittent Fasting, but is never recommended, not by anyone I've learnt from or read.

This is not because they don't have the same mission, but because you're expected to feed on some 'unketogenic' diets regularly when you are on intermittent fasting.

Those kinds of foods are legumes, vegs, grains and some oil.

Nobody would ever advise you to take alcohol or sugary foods on either diet plan, but on a regular scale, they are both diet plans and one says no to the other.

Now let's get you what you can eat when fasting intermittently.

Chapter 9: List of Fat Burning Foods.

Keegan, my colleague at the Health Spa noted in a recent interview that some people think they are fasting intermittently so they should lose pounds, but they keep feeding on f that returns triple of whatever pound they lost.

I don't want you to keep thinking you're trying my weight loss technique so you should be losing weight when in fact you eat meals that triple every lost pound.

If that happens, you think I gave wrong suggestions and you mix them with wrong dietary complications.

So, darling, find, mix and eat of the 20 goodies I am listing below.

a. Peas and Peanut Butter
b. Legumes: Black beans, Kidney Beans, Lentils and so on.
c. Rich Proteins: Chicken Breast, Scrambled Eggs, Beans, Greek Yoghurt, Meat, Shake, Eggs and so on.
d. Apples, avocados and Bananas.

e. Nuts

f.   Salmon and fatty fish.

g. Green Tea, Oolong Tea and Coffee.

h. Olive Oil, Coconut Oil and MCT Oil (That's got from coconut or palm oil, the store keepers have them a lot).

i. Tuna Fish

j. Unprocessed Grains.

k. Pumpkin

l.   Potato

m. Oats

n. Peas

o. Tomatoes and Onion

p. Chili

q. Citrus and Butternut Squash

r. Berries.

s.   Dairy

A bonus: Veggies, pastas and soups are allowed too.

Could I have missed your favorite?

I rarely do. You can eat them according to their nutrients content.

Try to get unprocessed ones too.

Chapter 10: Fasting Misconceptions

Now, let's see if you aren't making one of those mistakes most people make about intermittent fasting.

You are an expert already, and you probably can judge most of these questions. So, if you understand them well enough, you can tell the right answer to these wrong opinions people hold on Intermittent Fasting.

But don't get too excited. I think you'll be guilty of one at least. If you are, you pay by increasing your fasting window.

A deal? Let's go.

1. Intermittent Fasting Aids Eating Disorder: Does it? I'd argue anywhere that it doesn't. Intermittent Fasting helps you balance and regulate your food intake. There may be suggestions that you shouldn't skip a meal anytime. But who would subscribe to that kind of suggestion when it is having safety-threatening effects on them? Not me any way. By the way, Intermittent

Fasting doesn't cross out these suggestions, it allows you a stable and healthy body that can keep them going. In fact, OAU's publication believes that meals should be skipped once in a while and where does that leaves us? A goal in favor of Intermittent Fasting.

2. Intermittent Fasting Causes Starvations: No way, this isn't something I would take at all. Most busy people forget to eat already. Those who eat regularly understand that they need to move on empty bowel some times. In comparison with most other type of religious fasts that people engage in, Intermittent Fasting is lighter, and fun to try.

3. Intermittent Fasting tempts people to bulimia: no way! Well before you ask me, Bulimia is a state when people eat too much than they can contain and eventually vomit all again. Do we do that? No way, I remember one of the warnings I gave in that last page is that you just mustn't misuse your eating window and eat beyond what you can take in. Particularly because your calories are numbered, you can't take everything possible.

4. Your Performance reduces as an athlete: says who? I smile a lot when athletes walk to me and repeat this worry. Factually, eating less carbs can reduce your insulin levels which means energy reduces, but you would not doubt agree with me that intermittent Fasting means a lighter, faster and swifter body that can perform better in aerobic and anaerobic gamed. Which athletes doesn't need those powers? If you're worried about energy, calisthenics will always cover you up. Moreover, the easy Intermittent Fasting is so mild that you won't ever remember or feel your fast during training. Instead, some excess carbs that could have sat in your belly, inspired stomach aches or an unusually heavy body during sport is systematically cleared off the table.

5. Eating anything during eating Windows makes Intermittent Fasting Ineffective

I really believed this during my first few days of trying out intermittent fasting. Dr Roberts would always explain that no matter what you eat during your eating window, your body desires certain nutrients at certain times and your refusal to supply them during your fasting window means something, no matter how little, some pounds must drop off your body size on the scale. Eventually, I noticed that was true too.

6.Intermittent Fasting doesn't work for anyone: doesn't it? If you cut your coat to your size, why not? If you carefully look for the perfect plans considering your nature, it sure will work for you. Only the underweights, who do not need weight loss by default are exempted.

Take Away

You want to be a smart girl in America today? Your first task is to look smart. Dressing smartly will make you look nice, but you can imagine how it feels to look gorgeous naturally, then pluck into a smart dress.

At work, at club, at the party, at home, at the beach, at the beauty pageants', in the entertainment, academic and even athletic world, everywhere; check out the prettiest girls, they are always slender girls with exuberant curves. I don't think you should be an exception.

You also need to watch your weight because of some life-threatening complications than come hand in hand with obesity.

Research keep proving that slender girls live longer, they look 37 at 57 and 19 at 28. You shouldn't be an exception to that too. You may be fat already, and you may still be slim, but whatever it is, we all need to keep our body in shape.

Many methods may not work for you, and some would take your favorite diet far from you. That's exactly where Intermittent Fasting comes to the rescue.

You're in control of your weight and your diet.

I have listed many things you can gain by trying out Intermittent Fasting, I listed the bad sides too.

You'll find the various methods of Intermittent Fasting we have got in this book and I explained how you can calculate your chances of planning a perfect intermittent fasting being a busy woman, breastfeeding, menstruating, a sportswoman and one in her menopause.

I have listed the foods you can eat and those you should avoid during Intermittent Fasting.

I also tried telling you about Ketogenic diets in comparison with Intermittent Fasting. Remember learning about foods that can burn fats and misconceptions of people about intermittent fasting?

What else do you remember learning?

Have you picked a suitable intermittent fasting plan and you want some clarifications?

Feel free to go over this book again.

Hi, the newest smart lady in the States.